Controlling Your Weight

Getting Rid of the Chubbiness and Fat

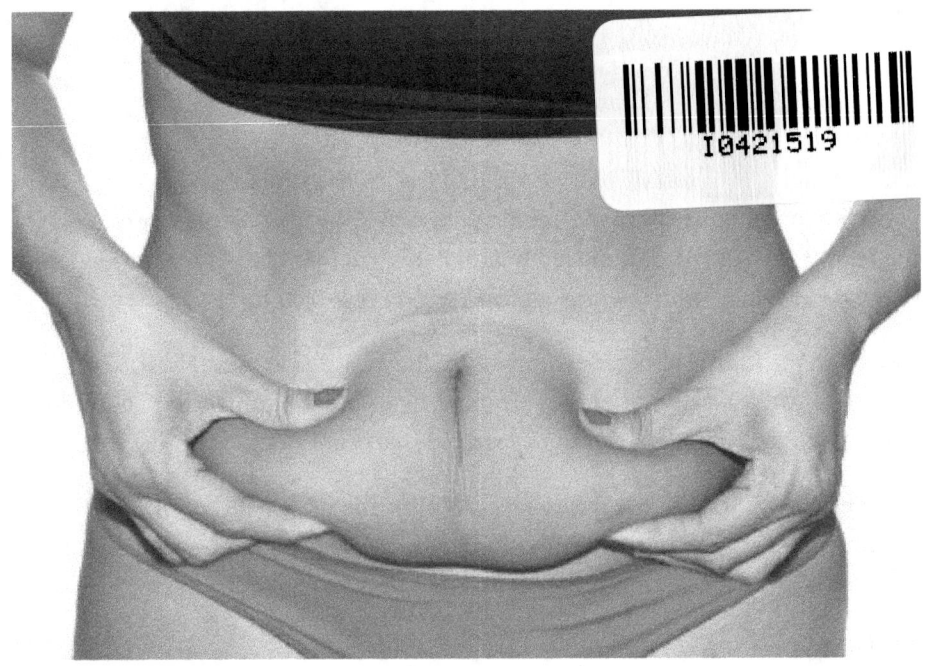

Dueep Jyot Singh

Mendon Cottage Books

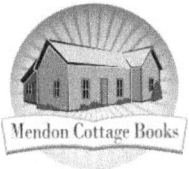

JD-Biz Publishing

Disclaimer

The information is this book is provided for informational purposes only. It is not intended to be used and medical advice or a substitute for proper medical treatment by a qualified health care provider. The information is believed to be accurate as presented based on research by the author.

The contents have not been evaluated by the U.S. Food and Drug Administration or any other Government or Health Organization and the contents in this book are not to be used to treat cure or prevent disease.

The author or publisher is not responsible for the use or safety of any diet, procedure or treatment mentioned in this book. The author or publisher is not responsible for errors or omissions that may exist.

Warning

The Book is for informational purposes only and before taking on any diet, treatment or medical procedure, it is recommended to consult with your primary health care provider.

Our books are available at

1. Amazon.com
2. Barnes and Noble
3. Itunes
4. Kobo
5. Smashwords
6. Google Play Books

Table of Contents

Introduction

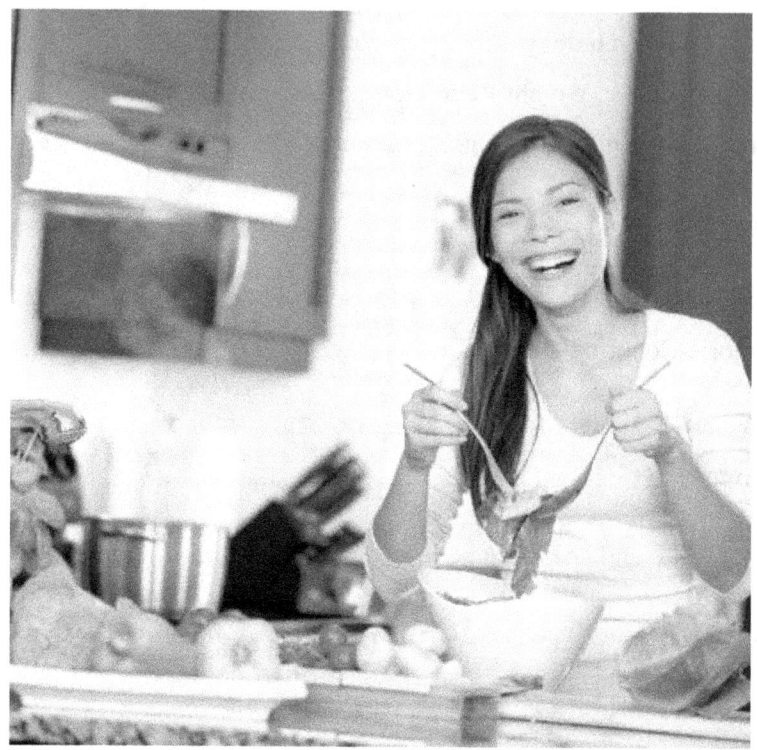

Healthy eating means a healthy body.

Just ask a number of your acquaintances out there, about their first priority in matters of health, and there is a chance that they are going to say that they are bothered about their increasing weight and how they can get rid of the fat accumulated on their bodies.

Naturally, thanks to social demands and the demands of fashion, all of us want a streamlined body. However, obsessing about a fashionably streamlined zero fat body is not something a normally sensible person should do or would do.

Remember that it is necessary for your body to have a little bit of fat present in it in order to keep functioning properly. Nature has provided you with fatty cells, under your skin in order to keep the skin in shape and to provide a cushion for the muscle, tissues and organs underneath. Also, this fat can be considered to be a reservoir which is going to provide your body with lots of energy in times of starvation.

The cells are going to be used by your liver to keep your body functioning properly, when you do not have enough of food to eat. Actually, this fatty layer was what saved human beings millenniums ago, when they needed to hunt for food and did not manage to capture that sabertooth or mastodon over a long period of time. This layer also protected them from freezing to death.

But nowadays, in the 20 first century, we do not need to go hunting for our daily lamb, or game. We have it easily accessible and that is why, instead of bothering about survival, we are more bothered about getting rid of all that ungainly fat, and our weight.

Incidentally, if you are well-rounded, like that famous comic character Obelix, you would not mind being called chubby. But you are immediately going to get indignant and annoyed, if anybody calls you fat. You may also describe yourself as Jovian, Amazonian, and well-rounded. And if you are an extra large size, you may wish that you were living in medieval times when well-rounded bodies and fat women were considered to be beautiful, as they were the symbol of the fertile mother Earth. Therefore, they were treasured, considered very attractive and also thus desirable.

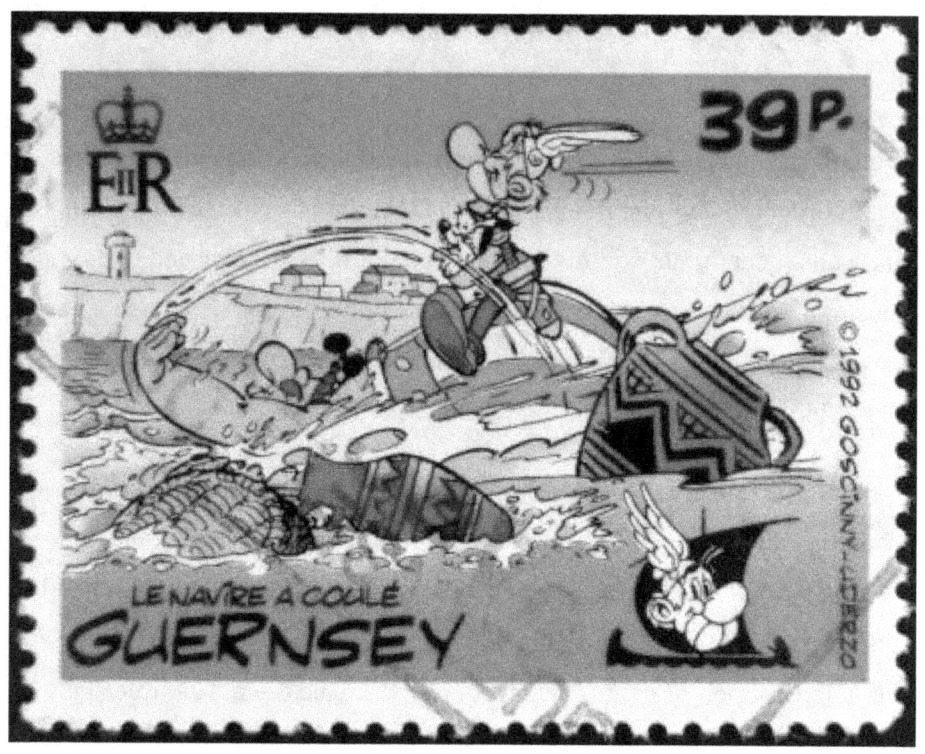

Obelix has never considered himself to be fat. He is well covered!

I Want to Be Thin…

Nevertheless, today, weight and dieting is one of the burning questions, which every health-conscious human being is concerned about. And as we are not living in a century where a woman who walked with the heavy step of an elephant, with solid busts and behinds were considered to be earth goddesses, we are more intent on being as thin as bamboo poles. So when did this concept of being as thin as a rake begin to hold sway on popular conscience and become one of the major demands of society?

First of all, take it as a mental set up, which began to be passed down from the ages, especially in Europe. Aristocrats considered women with big busts and behinds, large feet, and ungainly bodies to be peasants, "common" and plebeian.

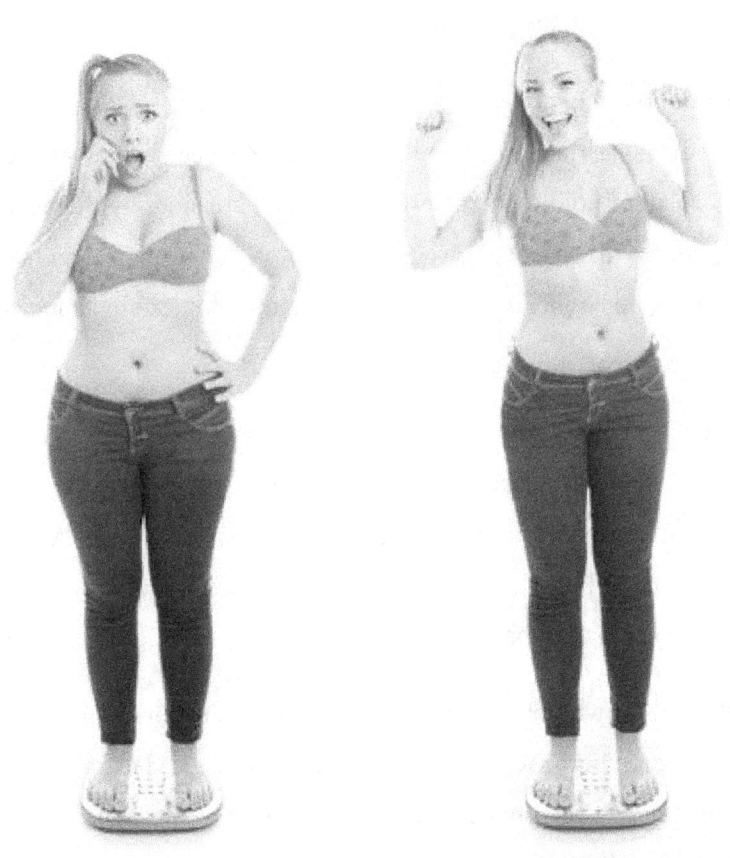

A true aristocrat was one who was thin, slim, with small hands and feet and with an arrogant patrician look. This was in ancient times. As time went by, people of "common blood" began to wish that they were genetically programmed in such a manner, that they could look like the slim, thin, and lean aristocrats.

And then came the first and the second world war. Due to a scarcity of food, everybody had reached the point of starvation. That is also when the social lines between "aristocrats" and "the oi polloi" began to be dissolved as something outdated, outmoded and not in keeping with the times.

Class distinction in many parts of Europe had begun to break down because both the world wars had equalized human beings because they needed to survive instead of holding themselves aloof and considering themselves of better blood! So that particular social revolution in Europe began to take the form of everyone having a slim, thin, almost anorexic, skeletal androgynous look.

And the idea that only those people could afford to be fat who managed to have enough of money to pay the black market dealers began to permeate in the social state of that time. So naturally, everybody wanted to be thin because this proved that they were patriotic! They starved with all their fellow countrymen and that showed on their bodies, and general health.

This is the reason why fashion designers began to encourage people to stay slim and skeletal, because after the wars, not many could afford to wear clothes, made for well-rounded and fat forms. One could either be extremely curvy and be totally and absolutely feminine or be that starved waif with not enough of food to eat. There were no in between stages of half rounded and half thin.

Weight and Psychology

Believe it or not, weight is an important factor which affects your psychology. A number of us are so geared to looking beautiful and attractive and that can only be achieved supposedly by being lean and thin, that we start suffering from low self-esteem, and loss of self-confidence.

In fact, many people who come to dietitians asking for weight reducing advice are normally teenagers. Surprisingly enough, teenagers begin to start worrying about their weight, either due to peer pressure, or possibly due to low self-esteem.

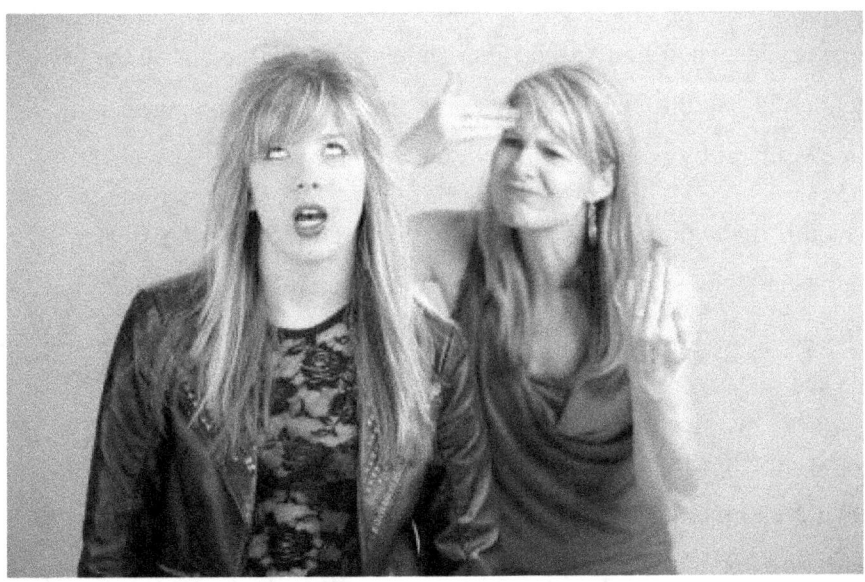

That is why they go to dietitians, asking for a strict regime with which they could lose their weight and become as slim and thin as either their favorite popstar or anyone else in their peer circle. If the dietitian is sensible, he is not going to encourage the teenager to think very much about their sudden gain in weight. This weight is because of the glands being overactive and this is soon going to pass so if you know anybody who is a teenager who thinks she is extra fat, ask her to cheer up. She is soon going to become streamlined in her twenties getting rid of all that puppy fat!

What do you mean you want body sculpting done because you are fat? You crazy or something?

This is the reason why so many women begin to suffer from anorexia or bulimia. Anorexia is a problem where people do not eat because they are afraid of getting fat. This means that they are going to the extreme. In severe cases, they starved themselves on purpose, or when they go on to an eating binge because their body needs nourishment, they purge out all the food by retching. Doing this continuously may harm the food canal, especially if you purge yourself by putting a finger down your throat.

I saw this being done by a teenager, who was thin to the point of starvation, but the cause she wanted to be a zero fat specimen like one of her favorite actresses, she stopped eating. And when she was starved, she had to eat, and then she underwent the feeling of guilt.

This young girl had to be hospitalized because she was suffering from dehydration, malnutrition, and had stopped eating food. So remember that this eating disorder is a dangerous condition and has to be treated both psychologically and practically.

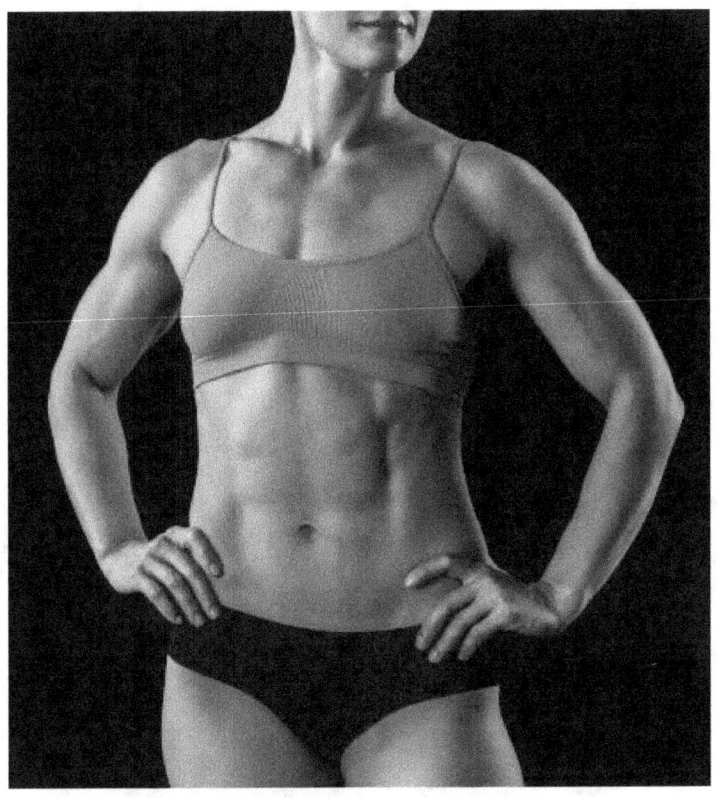

This is a zero fat condition in a female bodybuilder. Exercises have given her the feminine version of a six pack.

Many of us consider ourselves fortunate that we are mentally too strong to get into such an idiotic mental condition of not eating because we have let the topsy-turvy ideas of society influence us and thus play with our health. But that does not mean that a do not care attitude should make you say, what the heck, I am as I am, and if I am fat, so what. After all, it is my body.

One needs to think of weight reduction in the terms of how it is going to effect and influence our future state of health. Remember obesity can be potentially life-threatening because there are plenty of diseases which are caused or may be due to obesity.

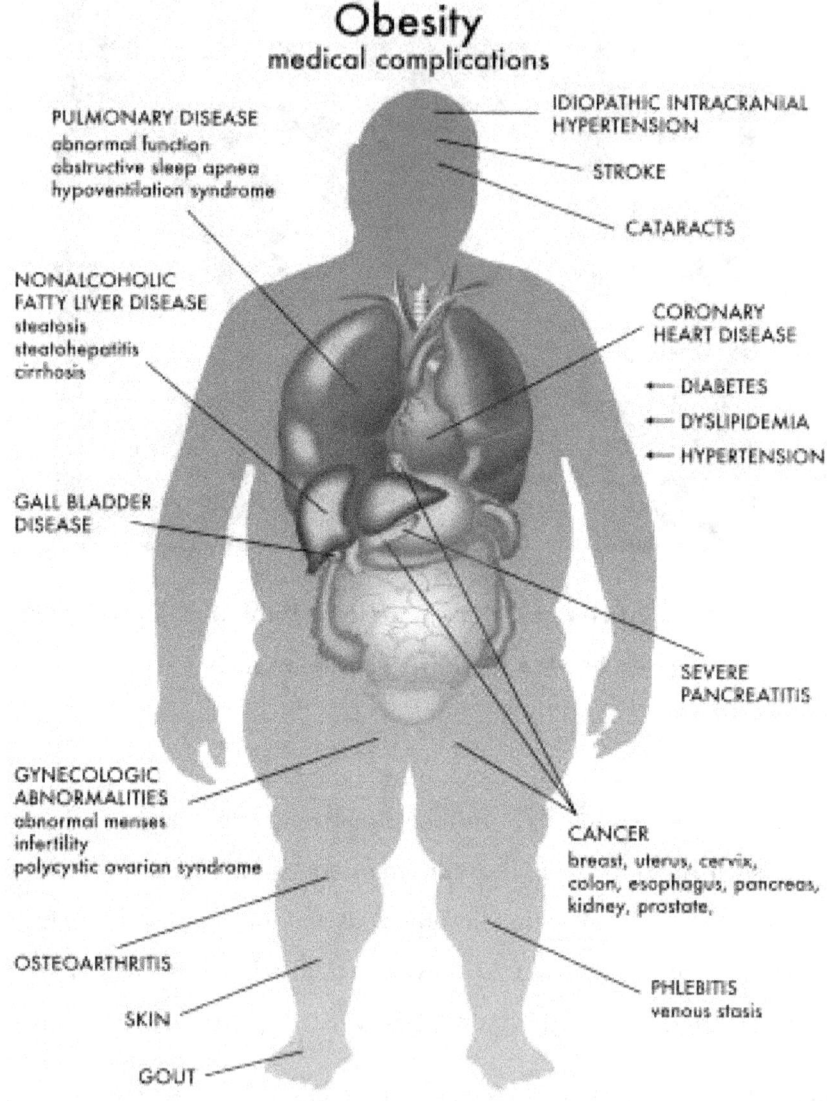

Obesity
medical complications

PULMONARY DISEASE
abnormal function
obstructive sleep apnea
hypoventilation syndrome

IDIOPATHIC INTRACRANIAL HYPERTENSION

STROKE

CATARACTS

NONALCOHOLIC FATTY LIVER DISEASE
steatosis
steatohepatitis
cirrhosis

CORONARY HEART DISEASE

DIABETES

DYSLIPIDEMIA

HYPERTENSION

GALL BLADDER DISEASE

SEVERE PANCREATITIS

GYNECOLOGIC ABNORMALITIES
abnormal menses
infertility
polycystic ovarian syndrome

CANCER
breast, uterus, cervix, colon, esophagus, pancreas, kidney, prostate,

OSTEOARTHRITIS

PHLEBITIS
venous stasis

SKIN

GOUT

Practical Tips for Weight Reduction

So here are some tips which you may want to follow, which are easily done with a little bit of self-discipline. These are practical tips and definitely do not include eating pills and medicines, which are supposedly going to make you lose fat overnight.

These tips are going to make certain that you never feel hungry. I do not intend that you should starve nor am I going to suggest any sort of drastic or crash diet. My intention is to keep you healthy while achieving your goal of weight reduction.

Do not eat between meals. I have seen a number of parents giving their children snacks in between meals, in order to keep them out of their hair and occupied. These children pick up the snacks and then go squat in front of the TV or the computer.

These parents are encouraging these children to follow a sedentary lifestyle. At the same time, they are stuffing them up like little geese with potato chips, and unhealthy junk food between meals. So these children are definitely going to suffer from a weight problem, as they grow older.

Not only are these snacks going to ruin your appetite, but they are also going to ruin your skin. Fried food items, vegetables like potatoes, pastries and cakes are definitely a no-no. However tempting they may be.

Also, it is not necessary for you to stop yourself to bursting point. Get up when you are still feeling a little bit hungry. Eat slowly and chew your food thoroughly. This is going to give you a feeling of "fullness."

Also, do not overload your plate. The more food you see on your plate, the more you would try to persuade yourself that you have to finish it up. But most of us are going to say, hey, this is too less, if we placed less amounts of food on our plate. This is a natural instinctive thought which comes into everybody's minds.

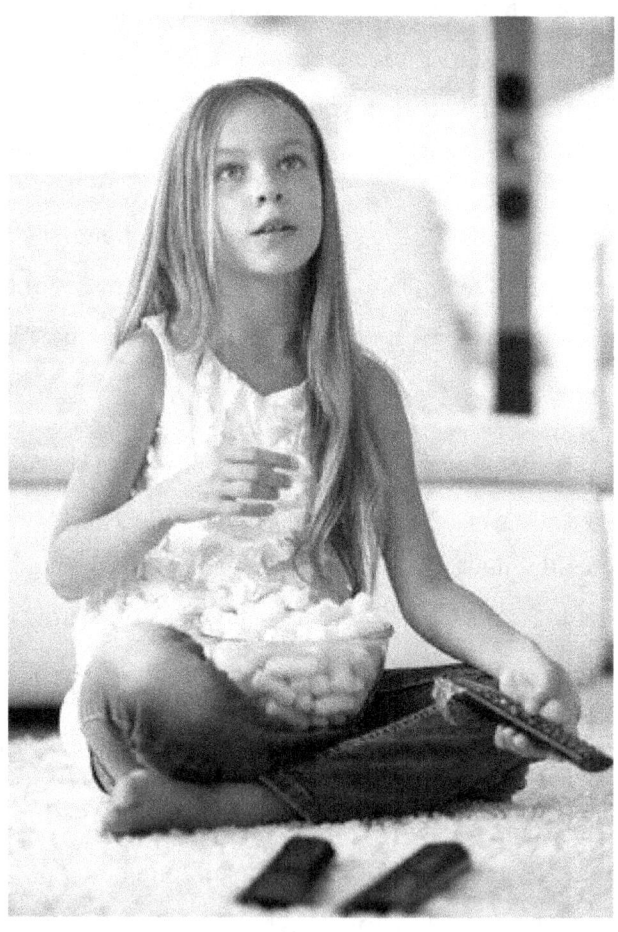

Do not worry about that. That is an instinct which has been inherited in human beings, down the ages. The wish is to fill our stomachs up, because who knows when we are going to get our next meal.

Luckily, we do not face that situation of potential starvation today. However, the instinct to fill up our plates is still there. And if you are trying to lose weight, this is definitely not something you would want to practice at every meal time.

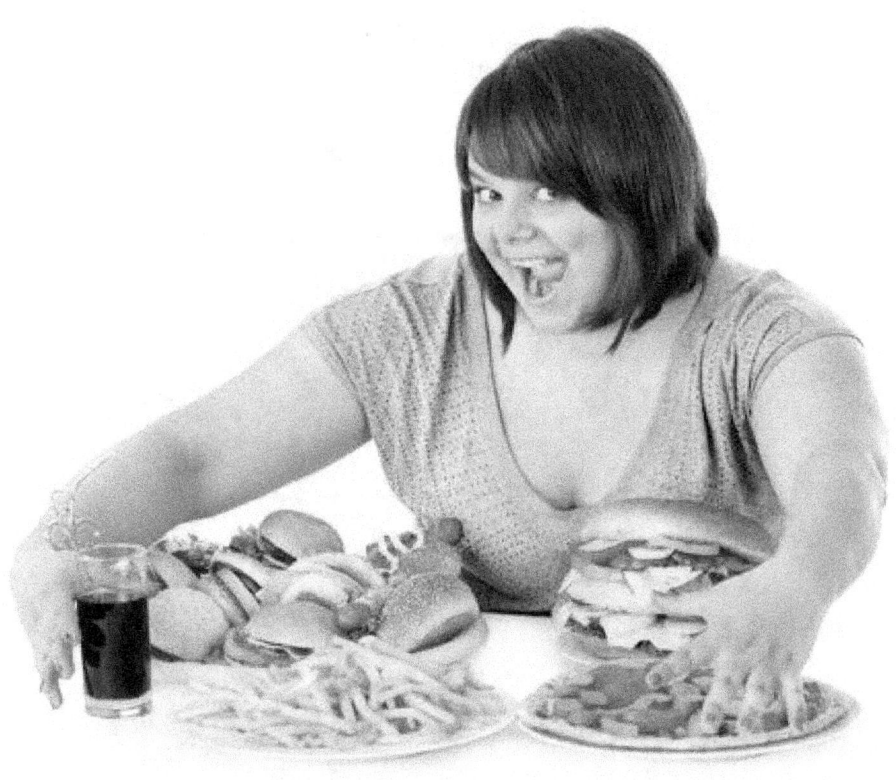

I would suggest using a half plate instead of a full-sized plate. So even if you overload it, you are going to be eating less than what you would be eating off a full-sized plate. Try this psychological trick.

Pick up the food items you want to eat. Spread them all over the plate in small portions. Fill up every inch of the plate. Your mind is immediately going to say, hey, the plate is full and now you can start eating.

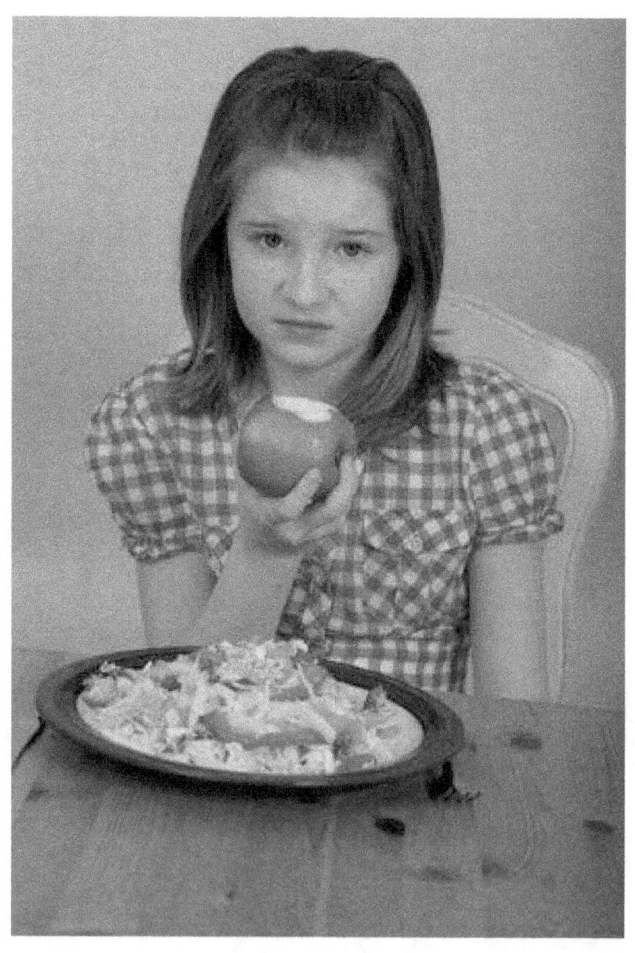

The mind has been visually notified that you have filled up your plate! And so it is satisfied.

I remember eating a gourmet meal, in a French restaurant, where the food was served beautifully decorated on our plates, but in really small portions. My French friends François and his wife Dominique appreciated it very much because they were used to eating small portions of food. After the meal was over, I thanked them for an excellent and delicious meal, came home and cooked a huge juicy steak!

My mind had not managed to persuade itself that that amount of food was adequate. Especially when one plate had just three mouthfuls. So your plate should have at least 6 to 7 mouthfuls. If you still feel that you are hungry, go back for seconds. However, those seconds should also be of minuscule amounts!

Talking about snacking and eating between meals. You may say do you practice what you preach, and I will have to reluctantly admit, that no, sometimes I do fall from this rule, especially when I am watching TV because at that time I need to keep munching something. So if you, like me, cannot resist snacking, you can satisfy that hunger with salads and fruit. Also dry fruit. I remember that too many dry fruit taken every single day may not be too good for your health, however much dietitians say that you should have lots and lots of them in your diet.

Take dry fruit in moderate quantities. Let me give you an example of the repercussions of these health giving food items when taken in large quantities.

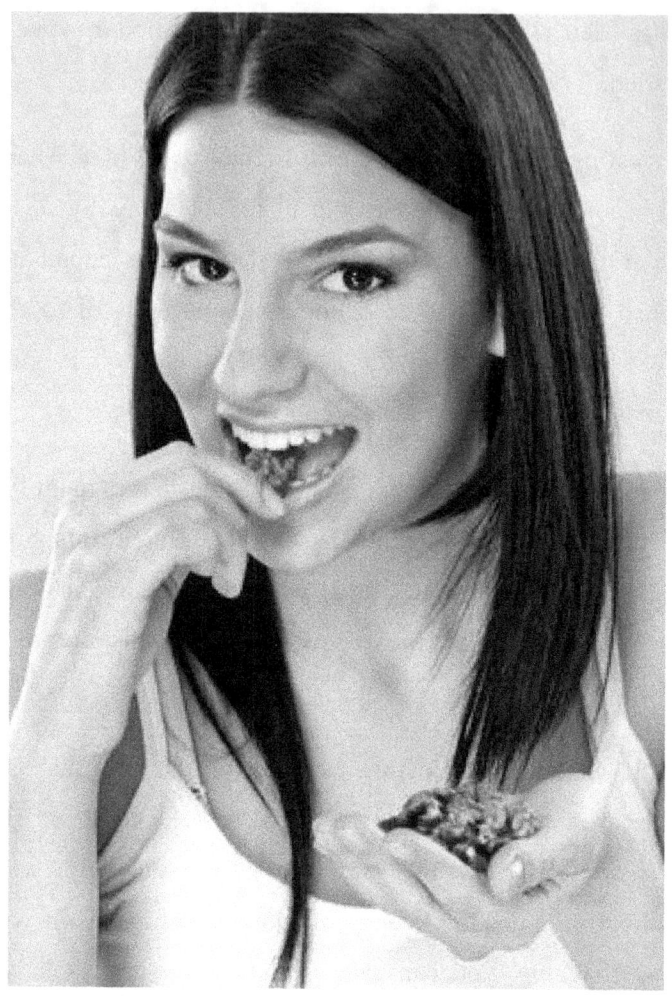

I was watching an interesting sports match, and I had some almonds at hand. By the time the match was finished, I had finished half a packet of these almonds, – about 20 of them. I still remember their activities during the night. Along with stomach pain, I had to go visit the bathroom often and that put me off almonds in any quantities for a number of years.

So remember that if you are engrossed in some particular sedentary visual activity, do remember what you are eating and how much.

The Bread-And-Butter Diet

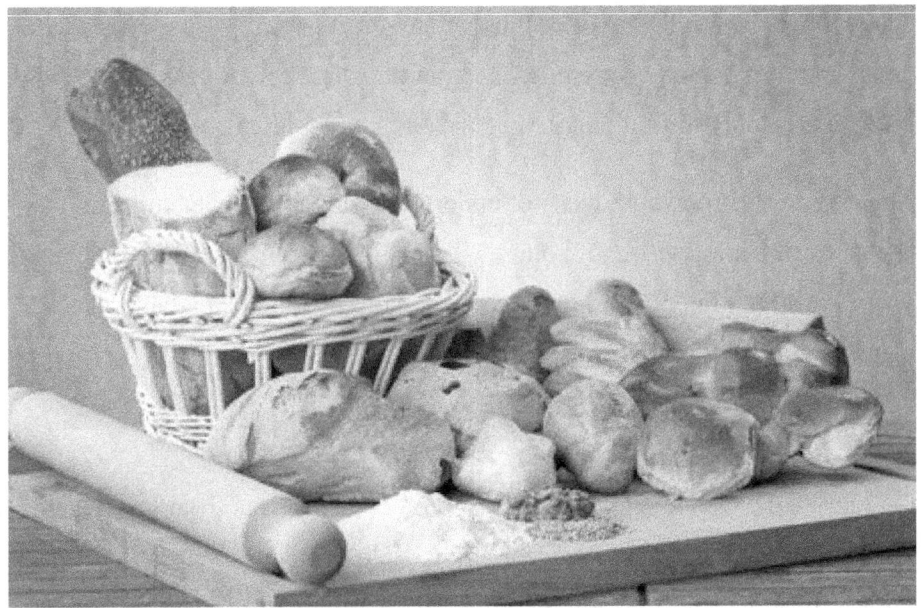

In the 1960s, a popular trend started up in the USA and in the UK. Women who wanted to lose weight began to undergo a bread and butter diet.[1] Is it possible to lose weight on such a diet? Yes, it is possible, but imagine needing four meals a day in which you are going to take a 400 g (one

---

[1] Bread and butter was in fact a child's diet, down the ages. In Beppo, the satirical Lord Byron says sarcastically – 'Tis true, your budding Miss is very charming/But shy and awkward at first coming out, /So much alarm'd, that she is quite alarming,/All Giggle, Blush--half Pertness, and half-Pout-- /And glancing at Mamma, for fear there's harm in /What you, she, it, or they, may be about; /The nursery still lisps out in all they utter--/Besides, they always smell of Bread and Butter.

pound) loaf of bread, 80 g (5 1/2 Tbsp) of butter, one glass of milk, and one glass of tomato juice. In the afternoon, you are going to drink weak tea with milk and one lump of sugar. Between meals, you can drink only water or barley water.

This is a really tough routine. But did you notice something here? There are absolutely no green leafy vegetables, or any meat proteins? There are the essential nutrients which are missing from this diet. So you may lose weight, but you are going to find yourself deprived of essential nutrients.

The body needs food and does not understand why you are submitting it to such a torture in the name of being fashionable and slim. If nature intended you to be streamlined, it would have made your metabolism adapt to such measures.

Genetics

Our ancestors needed a fat covering to protect themselves from the weather and also as a safeguard against starvation. But nowadays, getting rid of the fat is a full-time activity for many of us.

That is because many of us do not seem to understand that in a number of cases it is genetics which decides whether you are going to go through life looking like a cheetah or like a hippopotamus.

If your grandparents and parents were fat, how can you expect to look like Cindy Crawford or Naomi Campbell. Incidentally, these two ladies have kept their streamlined figures through rigorous dieting and also possibly through drugs.

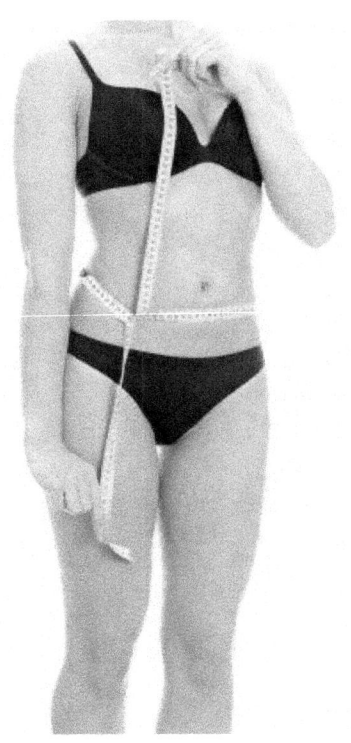

I want to have a waist like that of a supermodel...

You are definitely not going to be doing that. If you do not have Cindy Crawford's genes, you cannot expect to look like her. And if you came from a gene stock which was tubby, stocky and roly-poly, you cannot expect to be tall, slim, thin, however much you try to reduce, starve yourself or go on diets.

Sometimes thyroid gland secretions and problems can also cause extreme obesity or extreme thinness.

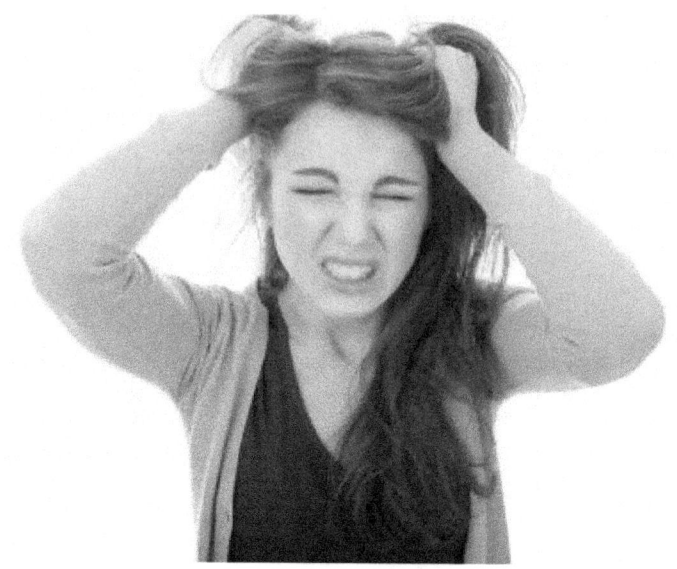

Do not get into such a state, ever, if you find yourself putting on weight. This process is natural as you grow older. And do not try to get rid of it, through starving yourself because society demands it.

Calories in Your Diet

Everybody keeps talking about calories, and how many do you normally need in your ordinary diet? Calories are the units of energy which are needed by your body in order to work effectively. A healthy person needs about 2000 cal per day and if you reduce your calorie intake to 1000 cal you are going to lose weight.

Like I said before, in the twentieth century and after the Two World Wars, the idea of being completely thin became an obsession. And that is why more and more folks stopped using healthy fat to cook food and instead started using chemical-based products or artificial products like margarine instead of natural foodstuffs.

Besides this, a caloric imbalance is the reason why people suffer from obesity and overweight. This means that you are expending too few calories in the form of "burning off calories" in proportion to the amounts of calories eaten in your diet. Also, environmental, behavioral, genetic and dietary factors are going to influence your health, possibly causing obesity and overweight problems.

You can find calories in butter, cheese, pastries and cakes, puddings, streets, sauces, soups, chocolate, cocoa, dried beans and dried fruit. For a low-calorie intake, you can eat spinach, green, fruit and salads, green leafy vegetables, etc.

Calorie Counting Diets

I was astonished to see a healthy 10-year-old girl making a diet chart of the calories taken in her meals, and weighing herself morning and night. When I asked her why she was doing so, she told me that her mother had told her that she was fat. Now, I have not come across a more blatant example of parental stupidity.

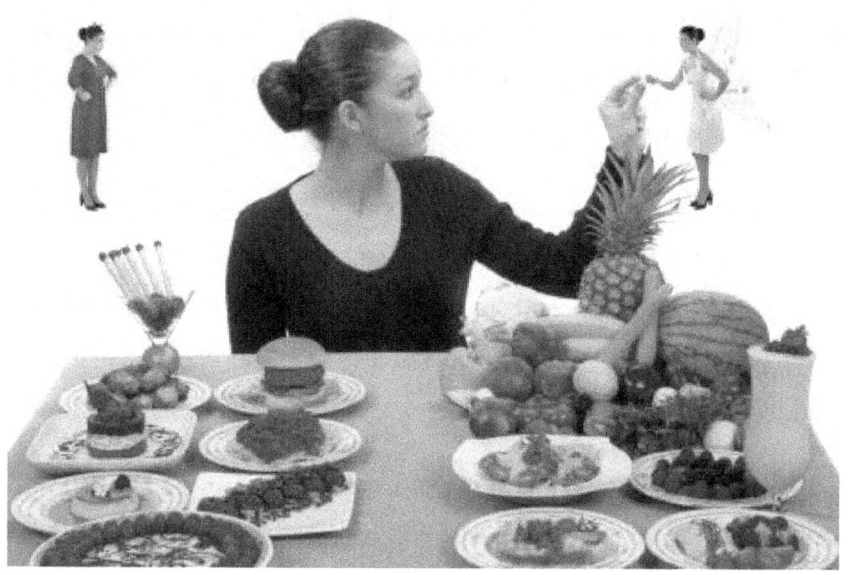

Not only is the mother causing her child to feel low self-esteem, but she has already set her on the way to future eating disorders.

Bulimia and anorexia are just harmful side effects of calorie counting diets. A 10-year-old child has absolutely no business counting calories, especially when she is a healthy child. Also, the idea of weighing herself morning and night is something psychologically abnormal.

But I knew the mother. She was obsessed with weight loss and weight gain. She was the first one to try out any diet, in the market and spent her paycheck on the latest weight-loss fad being followed by the stars. She was ruining her health steadily in an almost neurotic manner. And any diet that she followed had to be followed by the rest of the family, or else there is going to be World War III and pandemonium in the house.

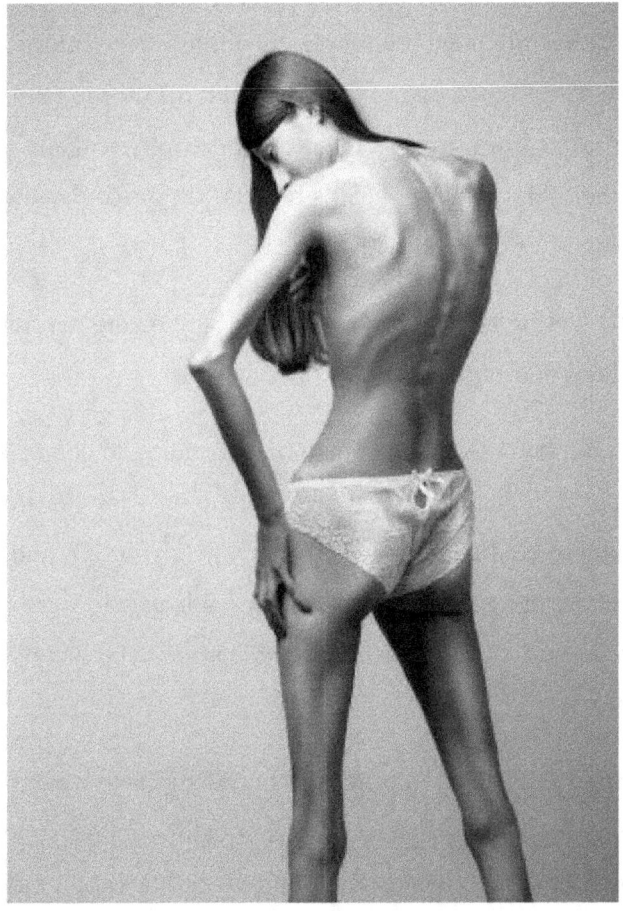

This looks horrible, but it is a reality. This young woman is suffering from a bad case of anorexia nervosa.

So now, thanks to her, her child had begun to obsess about weight loss and weight gain, at a very young age, when she should have been eating healthy nutritive meals in order to grow into a healthy adult.

Remember, obsessing about weight loss and weight gain to extremes is definitely not a healthy mental outlook. Counting every calorie eaten, and then worrying about how you are going to get it off, is one reason why so many people suffer from stress, tension and other physical and mental problems in their 20s and 30s. That is because they associate being slim and thin, with being physically attractive.

I know drastic dieting is the norm of the day, but you are depriving your body of essential nutrients.

What they do not know is that a human body is going to change as it ages. So your bio physiological and chemical makeup, in your 40s and 50s is definitely going to be different than what it was in your 20s and 30s. So if you think that you are going to be as slim and thin as you were in your 20s, when you are in your 50s, that is not possible unless you have been starving yourself regularly.

Calorie counting can keep you thin. But in order to lose weight or even maintain your weight, you have to keep your calorie intake so low that you are always going to feel hungry. Your body is on starvation mode and demands nutrition. You are not giving it proper nutrition. You are going to be sick continuously because your natural resistance and immunity system is all shot to pieces.

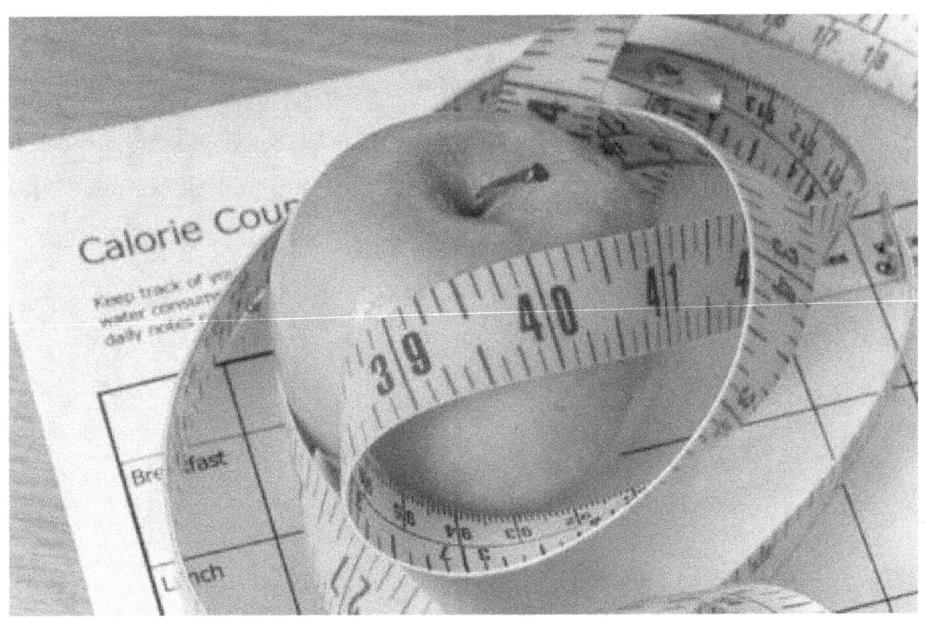

You are not going to have any resistance to disease. You are going to take 3 times as long as anyone else to heal, when you are sick and you are always going to feel weak and tired. Do you think this is worth the prospective chance of being ill forever more in order to look as skeletal as Victoria Beckham? I do not think so.

Besides this, you are also going to suffer from low blood sugar or hypoglycemia, because you are walking around hungry. Do not blame me if one fine day, you collapse, and have to be hospitalized because you are suffering from malnutrition and the accompanying diseases brought about through this slow starvation.

Also remember that the damage done during the starvation years are never quite going to go away. You are always going to suffer from ill health, in the future.

Look at the celebrities who are gaining proper popularity in the media with their zero fat figures. Why are so many famous stars hiding signs of ill health, brought on by starvation? That is because their managers did not bother to tell them that all those diets were doing harm to their bodies. All those tantrums and prima Donna acts thrown by stars can be avoided if they are caught by the scruff of their necks and fed good healthy, nutritious meals.

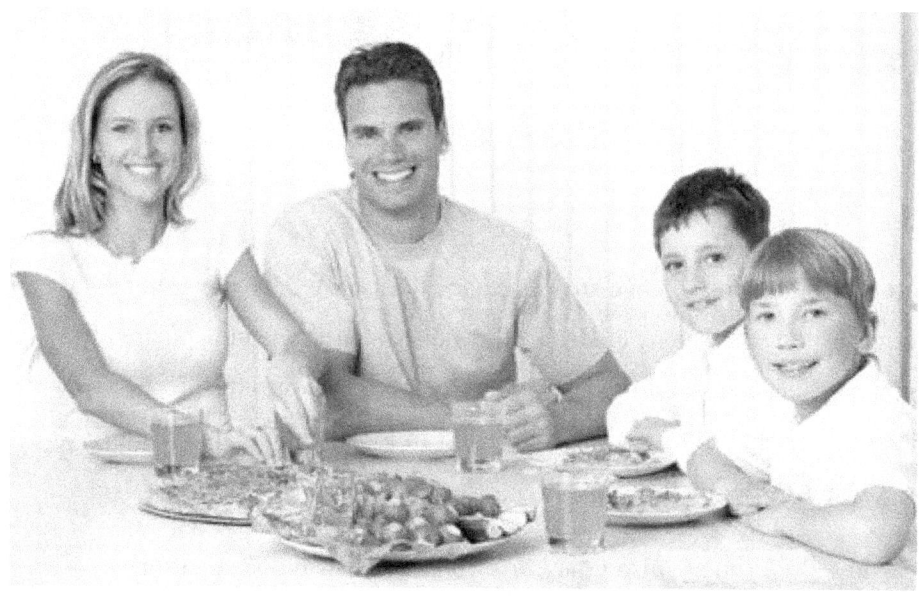

A healthy diet means a healthy family.

That is because low blood sugar means low energy levels. It also means bad temper, loss of concentration, and a muzzy outlook towards the world and your surroundings.

If you strictly restrict calories throughout your life, you are not going to get enough nutrition to keep you healthy. So for all those people counting calories, stop doing that, if you are basically a healthy person. It is only when your doctor asks you to watch your calories because you are suffering from some ailment and a restricted diet is necessary to heal your problem, that you need to follow his advice.

Exercises for Weight Loss

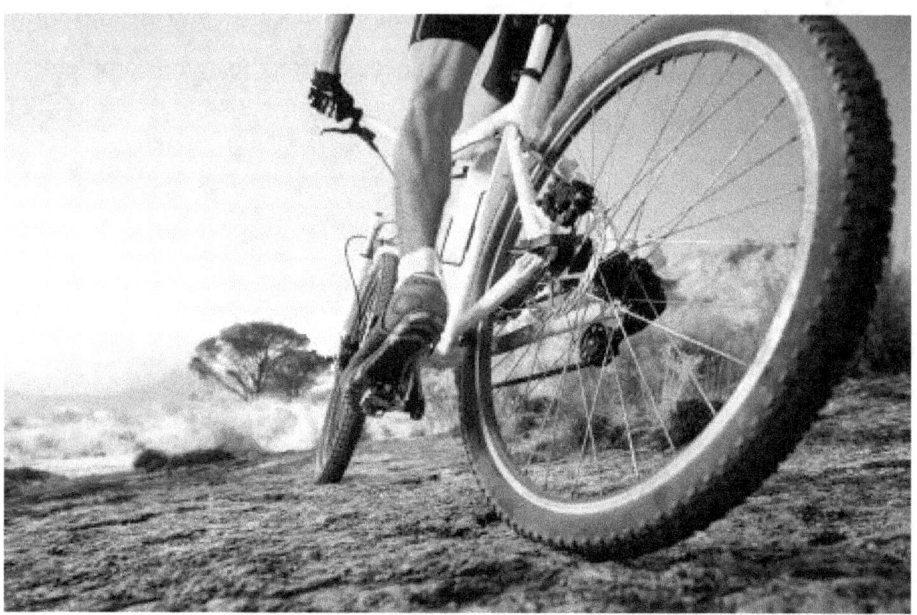

Cycling is a muscle development exercise. It does not help you get rid of fat from the leg and thigh regions.

I heard a colleague one say that exercising like cycling could make her fat legs turn slim and trim. She was annoyed with me when I said no, that exercise would make matters worse. So for all those people who think that cycling is going to reduce the fat from the legs, the answer is in the negative.

Cycling is a muscle developing exercise. Even swimming and dancing is going to aggravate matters!

Exercises under two headings – reducing and development. People used to think that if you drink plenty of water, you would become slim but sometimes it does exactly the opposite. You retain water and that makes up fat.

In fact, drinking up 8 to 10 glasses of water and then wondering by your ankles were so swollen up meant that you were suffering both from dehydration and water retention. In such cases you need to stop taking salt and put your feet up whenever you rest.

But as we are talking about weight reducing exercises instead of muscle development exercises, here are some tips. Exercise should never be treated as a duty of getting it over with because you have to do it every day. You need to make it enjoyable. Put on some music and some loose clothing. Fresh air is important so do your exercise in front of an open window. Do not hold your breath while exercising.

Stomach Exercises

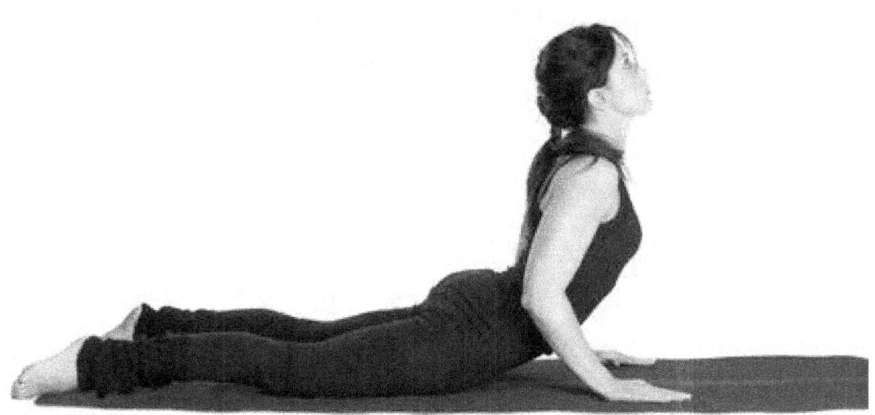

This exercise is excellent for your waist and stomach.

Usual and normal Stomach exercises are normally not muscular development exercises, unless you are into developing a six pack. They are going to help in reducing the fat content around your waist and firming it.

You need to learn how to brace it, in and up. Make sure that your stomach does not sag like as if you are dropping it in a bag at the bottom of your stomach!

Models have a practiced way of walking. The stomach is in and the behind is in. This is an exercise in itself. Do not walk with your shoulders hunched.

Your stomach should be up and in and your hips should be slightly forward. Also while walking, take a deep breath and pull your stomach muscles in. Exhale slowly but do not let your stomach out. This is to remind you that your stomach should be in when you are walking and not sagging all over the place.

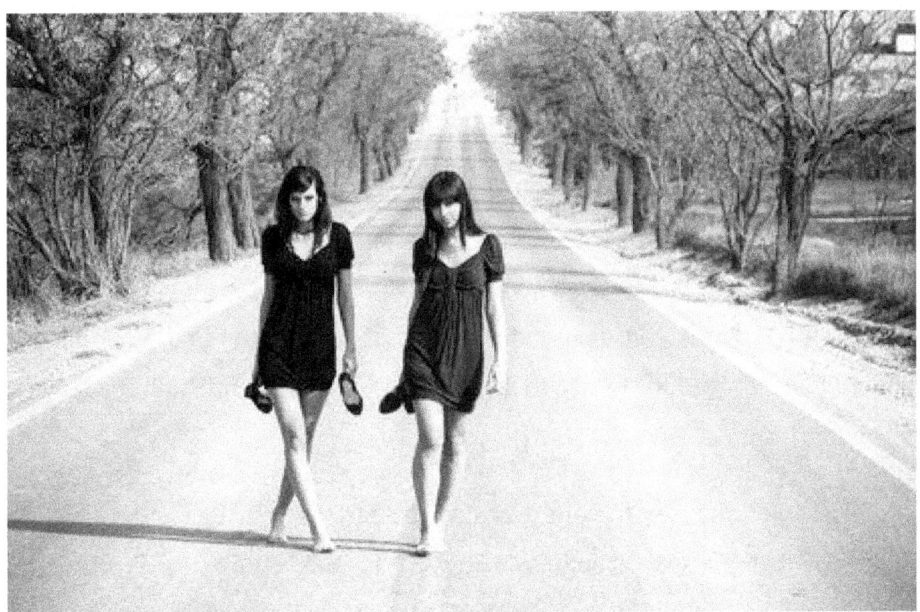

This particular walk, especially when you are walking from your hips, with one foot in front of the other is going to be successful only when you have tucked in your stomach.

Sometimes you may stand before your bathroom mirror, then you are washing your face or doing any other activity that is when you can see the pull in your stomach muscles playing on the abdominal muscles. Learn to do this automatically.

Now you may say that it is tiring, lifting up your stomach like that. Of course it is going to be tiring in the initial stages because you are not used to using those particular muscles but when it becomes second nature, it is to become easier.

Here are some more stomach exercises –

Lie flat breathing deeply in and out. Divide each breath into three little jerks for your stomach in at each little jerk. Let your breath out without bulging your stomach. Do this in a couple of groups of six with a good rest in between.

Lie down flat. Hook your feet under a piece of furniture and put your hands under the head, then try to rise to a sitting position without lifting the feet from the floor.

Lie flat on your back with your legs straight. Stretch your feet and rotate them slowly. Now slowly begin raising your head, keeping your knee still straight and bend your head slowly towards the knees. This is of course a very "painful" exercise, but it is going to get rid of that extra waist fat, really effectively.

Don't do this exercise in jerky movements. Now try to touch your forehead to your knees. At the same time, your elbows should be slightly bent and should be placed under your knees, in order to support them. Do this 3 to 4 times in the initial stages, until you can manage to press your head against your knees with the passing of time.

Spare Tire and an Obese behind

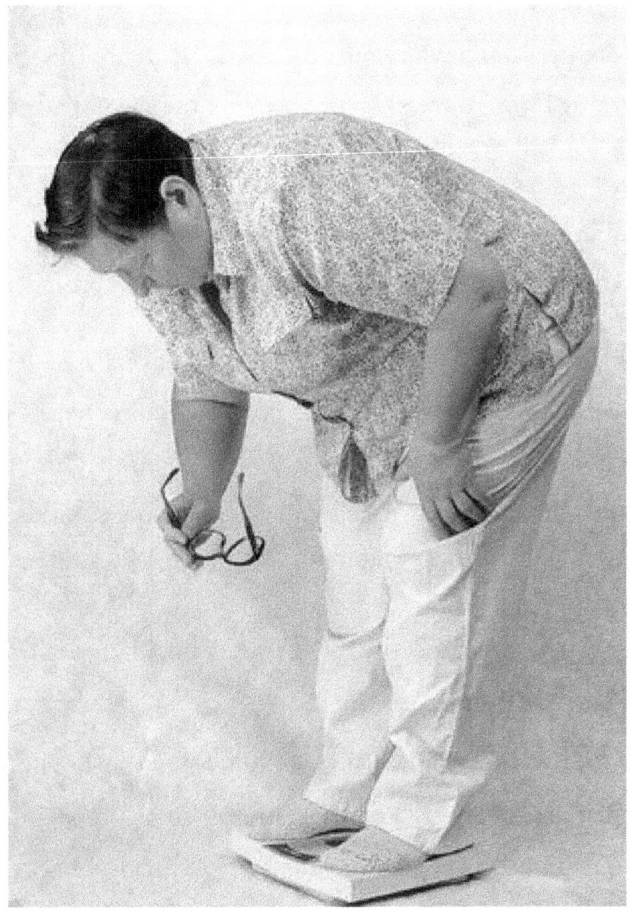

The moment we reach our thirties and forties, we begin to obsess about our spare tires, and also an obese behind in the case of many women. Like I said before, we are not in the medieval times, when Botticelli and Rubens would have gone gaga over our full figures and immortalized it on canvas.

So if you have a behind which bulges a bit, all you have to do is lie down with your toes pressed against the wall. Then contract your seat muscles. This is going to help in reducing the size of your behind.

As for the spare tire, stand with your feet apart and your arms under your hips. Lean forward from the waist only keeping the lower part of the torso stiff.

Swing around in big circles pulling at the waist. The whole spare tire has to move around and thus it is going to decide to reduce accordingly!

Also, it is very difficult to touch your toes, if you have a spare tire in between. Nevertheless, you may want to do this exercise nearly a dozen times everyday in just one easy step. Keep your knee stiff, lift up your hands. Swinging down quickly touch your toes without bending your knees. But make sure there is no quick and abrupt movement which puts a strain upon your back.

Hip and Thigh Exercises

If you are worried about your ever-expanding hips, crouch with your arms hunched about your knees. This position looks like as if you are getting ready to run a marathon. Then sway your body to and fro, backwards and forwards, with emphasis on the leg muscles.

You can also lie face down on the floor with your chin resting on the back of your hands. Then slowly lift your head up from the ground which is quite difficult because at the same time you are trying to lift up your legs, one at a time, also! Do this very slowly.

As for the rather crudely termed thunder thighs which look nasty instead of tasty, here is a nasty dose of exercises to get rid of them. They are tiresome, but they are extremely effective.

Lie on your back and double your knees to your chest.

Keep your feet together. Then shoot both the legs about to your right then slowly pendulum wise, rotate your legs to the left and then to the original position again. Rotate your legs this way about eight times to each side.

Rest for a minute, and then do some air by cycling with your self still lying down. When my friend who is an exercise instructor told me this, and use the example of a baby rotating its legs, I had to tell her that the baby had about four decades advantage over a flexible body, than I had! Besides, it could put its toes in its mouth or touch its face with its toes and there was no question of my doing that, however much she thought it a good stomach reducing exercise! I did not intend to twist myself into a pretzel form. So here is another easy way in which you can reduce the fat content about your thighs.

Stand straight, swing and touch your toes left right left right. This is good for your waist and it is also good for your thighs. I told you this exercise for your waist, above.

Waist Exercises

A friend of mine was admiring Jayne Mansfield's hourglass figure, and as I have the habit of raining on everybody's parade, I told her that these proportions were abnormal, natural and unhealthy. The thin waist which can be spanned by a man's hand, in Victorian times was because of these women cinching up their waists in tight whalebone corsets.

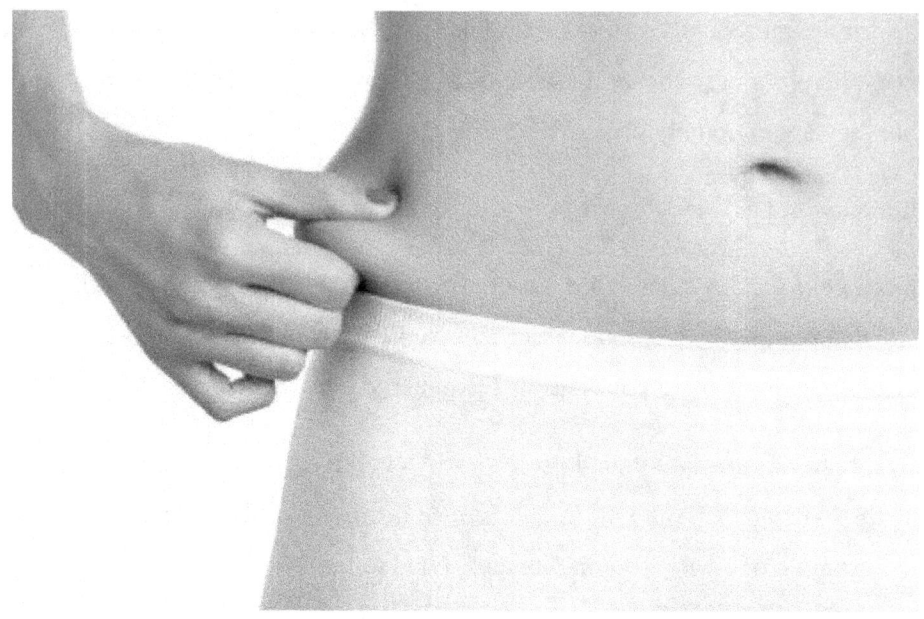

Even in Gone with the Wind, Scarlett O'Hara had to be laced in these tight corsets, so that she could have that tiny waist whenever she went into public. And that is the reason why these females kept fainting all over the place because their lungs did not get enough of air. And the men around them considered them to be really delicate and fragile lilies, when confronted with anything which disturbed their sensitive sensibilities.

A person who has the ideal hourglass figure is going to look lopsided, heavy up and down and nothing in the middle. They are going to totter and teeter because their center of gravity is all messed up.

However, as we are concentrating on getting rid of that extra fat around our waist and pelvic regions, just lie down on the floor with the arms stretched straight above the head.

Then pulled the knees up to the chest and rolled over to the left side so that their rest on the floor. Then slowly roll your knees over to the right side with your body still facing left!

This is going to put a twist in the waistline. You have to feel that twist and pressure. After that, stand with your feet apart, with your arms outstretched or level with the shoulders.

Twist from the waist as far around to the left as you can. Stretch down and grasped the left calf with your right hand. Repeat this by going for one side to the other side.

Now stand with your feet apart. Bend well ahead and forward with your arms hanging loosely like that of a ragdoll. Now turn your body from the waist around to the left, then smartly round to the right, swinging your arms and your whole body as you wish. Do this exercise 10 times.

Conclusion

This book is for all those people who are worried about their weight and want to find ways of reducing and controlling it. Remember that there is absolutely no shortcut in the world, which can cause you to lose weight overnight. If this happens, there is a chance that you are suffering from some sort of dread ailment. Drastic weight loss is not a healthy sign and you will need to go to a doctor for a complete medical checkup.

You need a little bit of body fat in order to keep healthy. You may be genetically inclined to fat, but looking at the people around you, you intend to be as thin, and slim as a streamlined panther.

People are definitely not happy with what they have and they keep on dreaming of the grass which is greener on the other side of the fence. This grass includes something more perfect to gain the approval of a society predominantly made up of outmoded and outdated concepts. These include huge busts which would make a female look like an original Jersey cow.

Also, men do not escape this sort of societal demands. They have to have zero fat waists, a muscular physique and other masculine attributes, which according to society are necessary to make them look attractive, macho and an all round He-Man.

This is the reason why so many people get caught up by conmen offering them magic, lotions, potions, and pills which are going to reduce weight. These pills may have diuretics in them which is going to get rid of all the water retained in your body. And you are pleased, because according to you, you have lost weight. Unfortunately, this weight loss is temporary, and as long as you are eating a proper diet, you are going to find yourself putting this weight on again.

So do not go in for any sort of weight loss fads which demand that you starve your body of essential nutrients. Also, detoxification diets are not healthy, especially if you are eating a mixture made up of red capsicum powder and maple syrup! Where is the nutrient content in this horrible mixture? But in the fifties, it was one of the most popular detoxification diets started up by a quack who called himself a doctor.

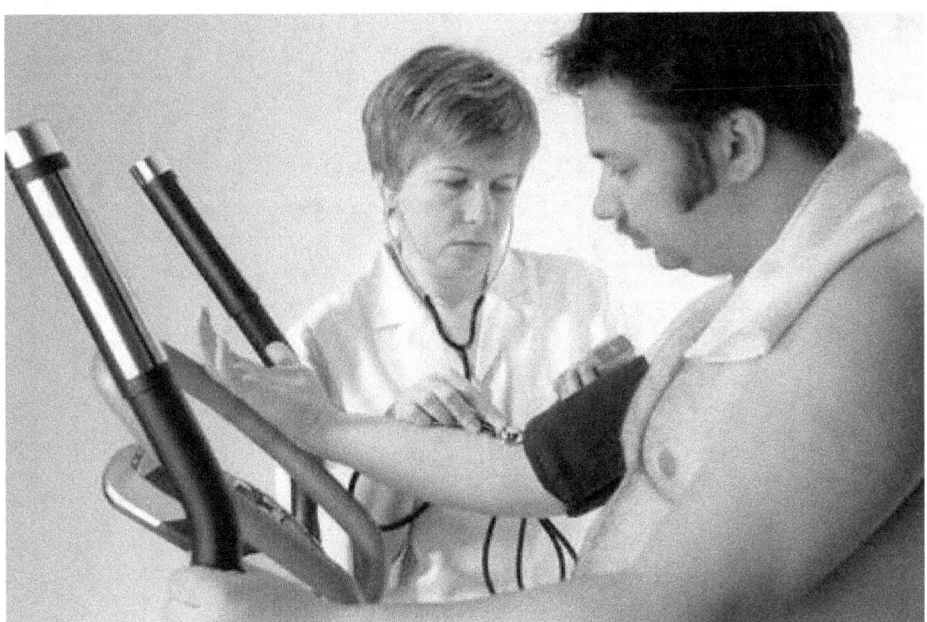

So be sensible about how you decide to lose weight. Weight loss is going to be a gradual process. If you lose about 4 pounds in about two months, it is going to be a healthy trend, because that means your body is customizing itself to manage in a healthy fashion, without that extra poundage.

So remember, no starvation, no drastic diets, and if you find yourself uncomfortable when doing exercises, and your body subjected to some sort of painful trauma, discontinue the exercises immediately!

Live Long, Live Healthy and Prosper!

Author Bio

Dueep Jyot Singh is a Management and IT Professional who managed to gather Postgraduate qualifications in Management and English and Degrees in Science, French and Education while pursuing different enjoyable career options like being an hospital administrator, IT,SEO and HRD Database Manager/ trainer, movie , radio and TV scriptwriter, theatre artiste and public speaker, lecturer in French, Marketing and Advertising, ex-Editor of Hearts On Fire (now known as Solstice) Books Missouri USA, advice columnist and cartoonist, publisher and Aviation School trainer, ex-moderator on Medico.in, banker, student councilor ,travelogue writer … among other things!

One fine morning, she decided that she had enough of killing herself by Degrees and went back to her first love -- writing. It's more enjoyable! She already has 48 published academic and 14 fiction- in- different- genre books under her belt.

When she is not designing websites or making Graphic design illustrations for clients , she is browsing through old bookshops hunting for treasures, of which she has an enviable collection – including R.L. Stevenson, O.Henry, Dornford Yates, Maurice Walsh, De Maupassant, Victor Hugo, Sapper, C.N. Williamson, "Bartimeus" and the crown of her collection- Dickens "The Old Curiosity Shop," and "Martin Chuzzlewit" and so on… Just call her "Renaissance Woman") - collecting herbal remedies, acting like Universal Helping Hand/Agony Aunt, or escaping to her dear mountains for a bit of exploring, collecting herbs and plants and trekking.

Check out some of the other JD-Biz Publishing books

Gardening Series on Amazon

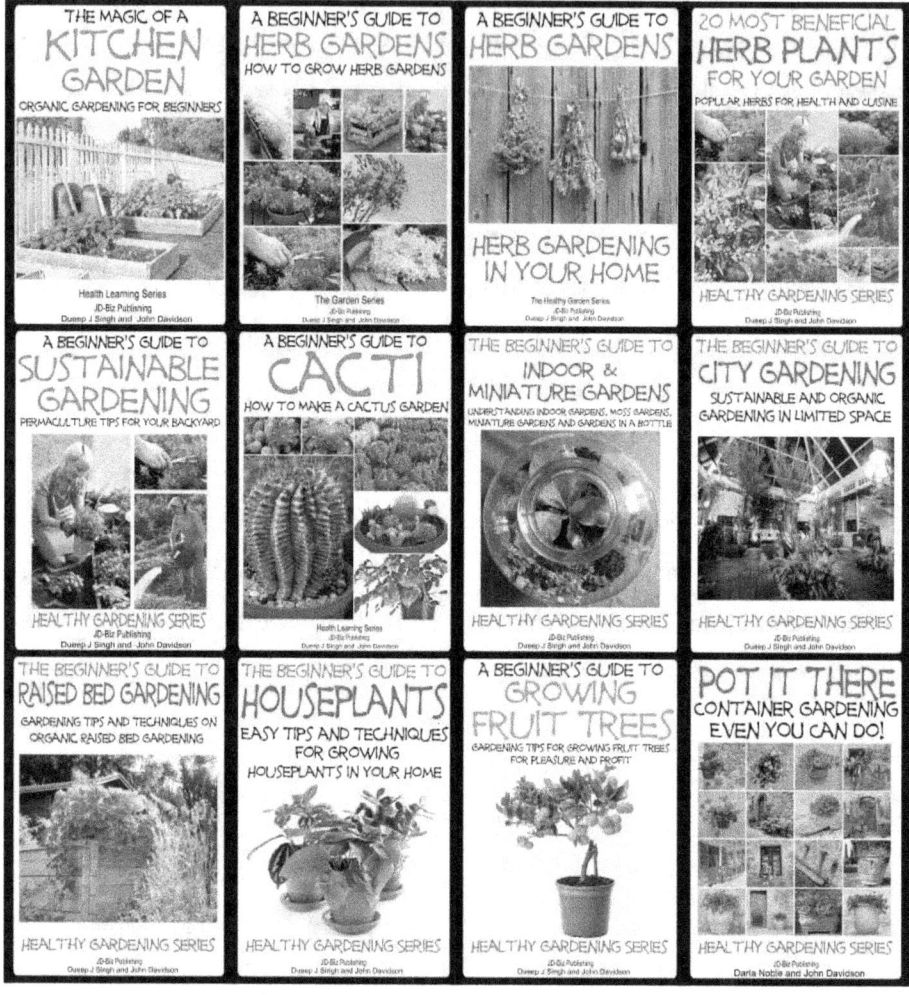

Health Learning Series

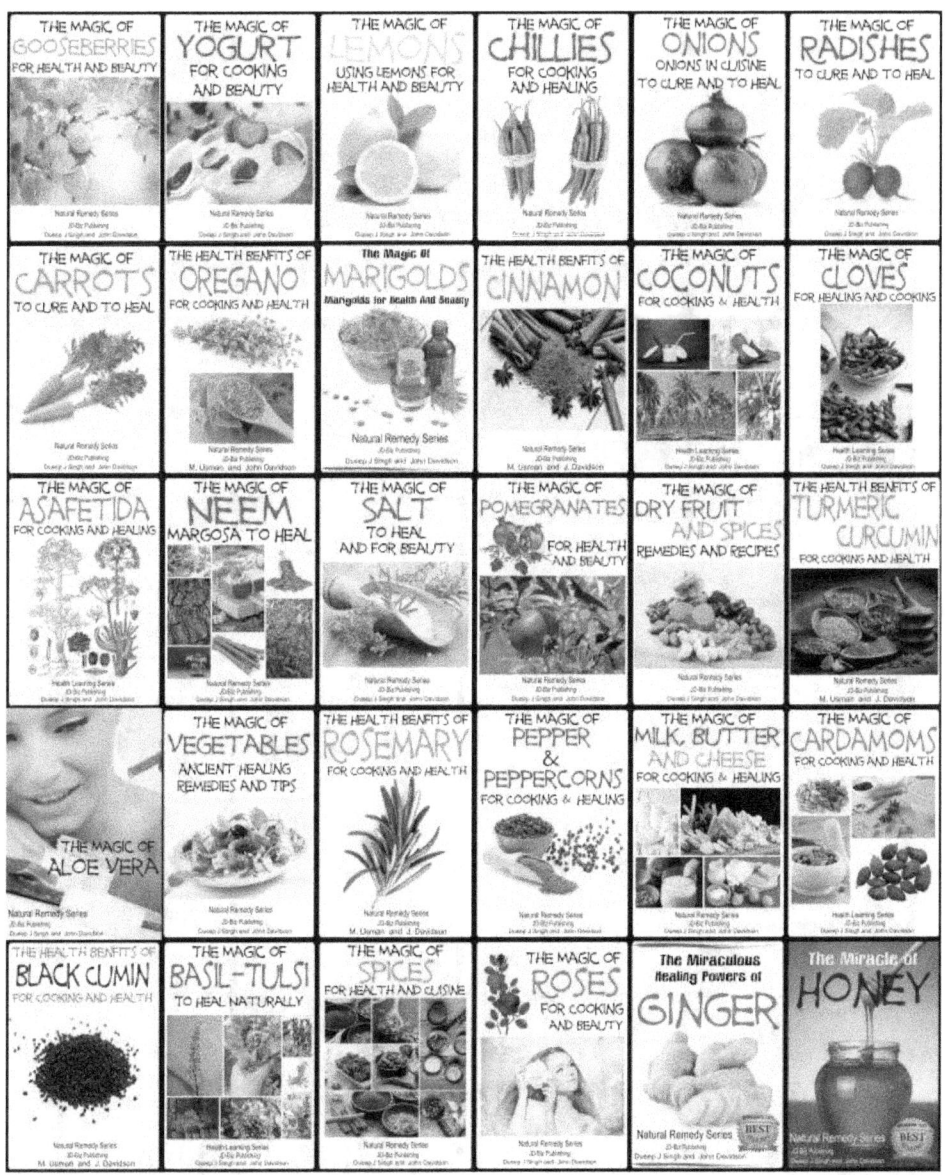

Country Life Books

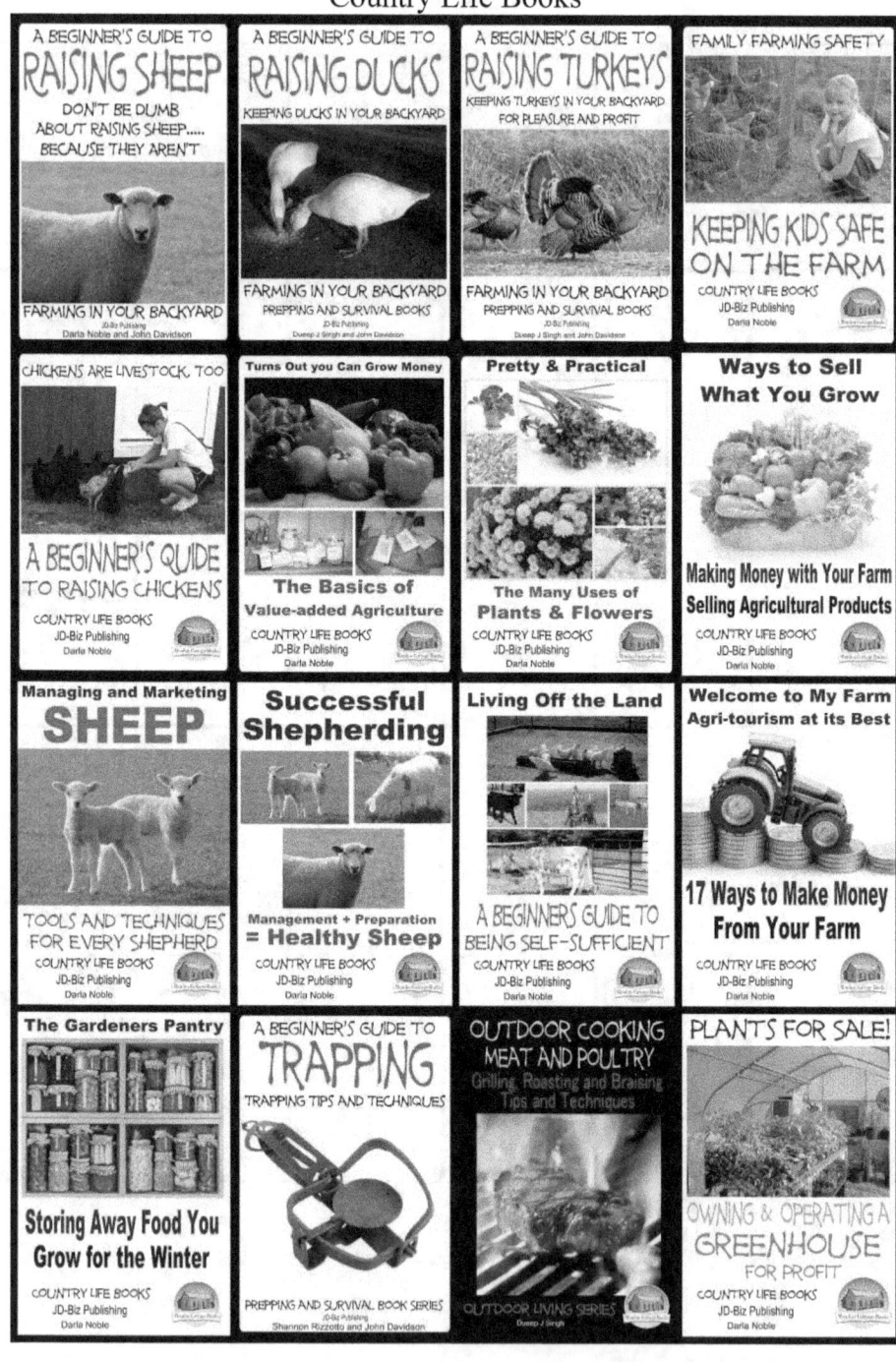

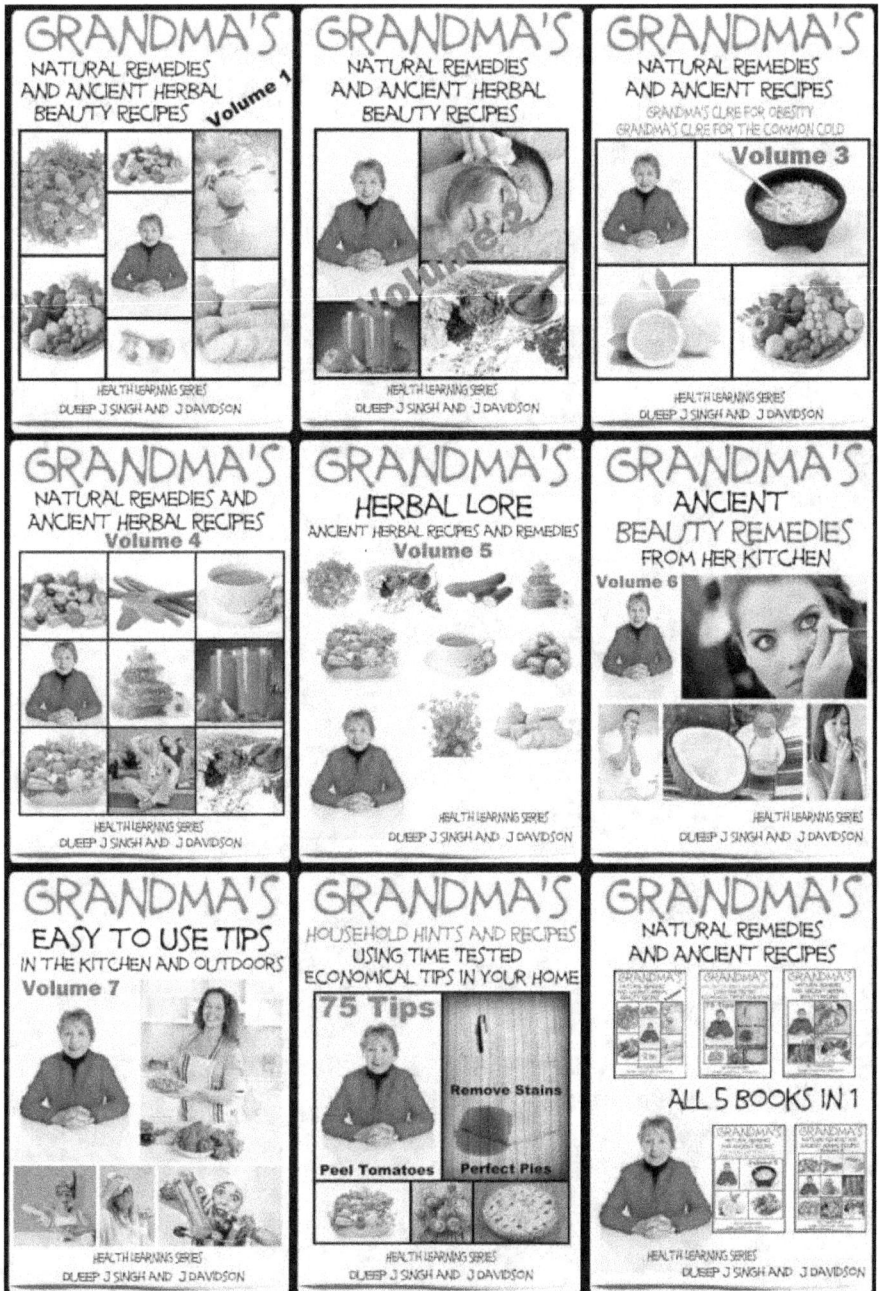

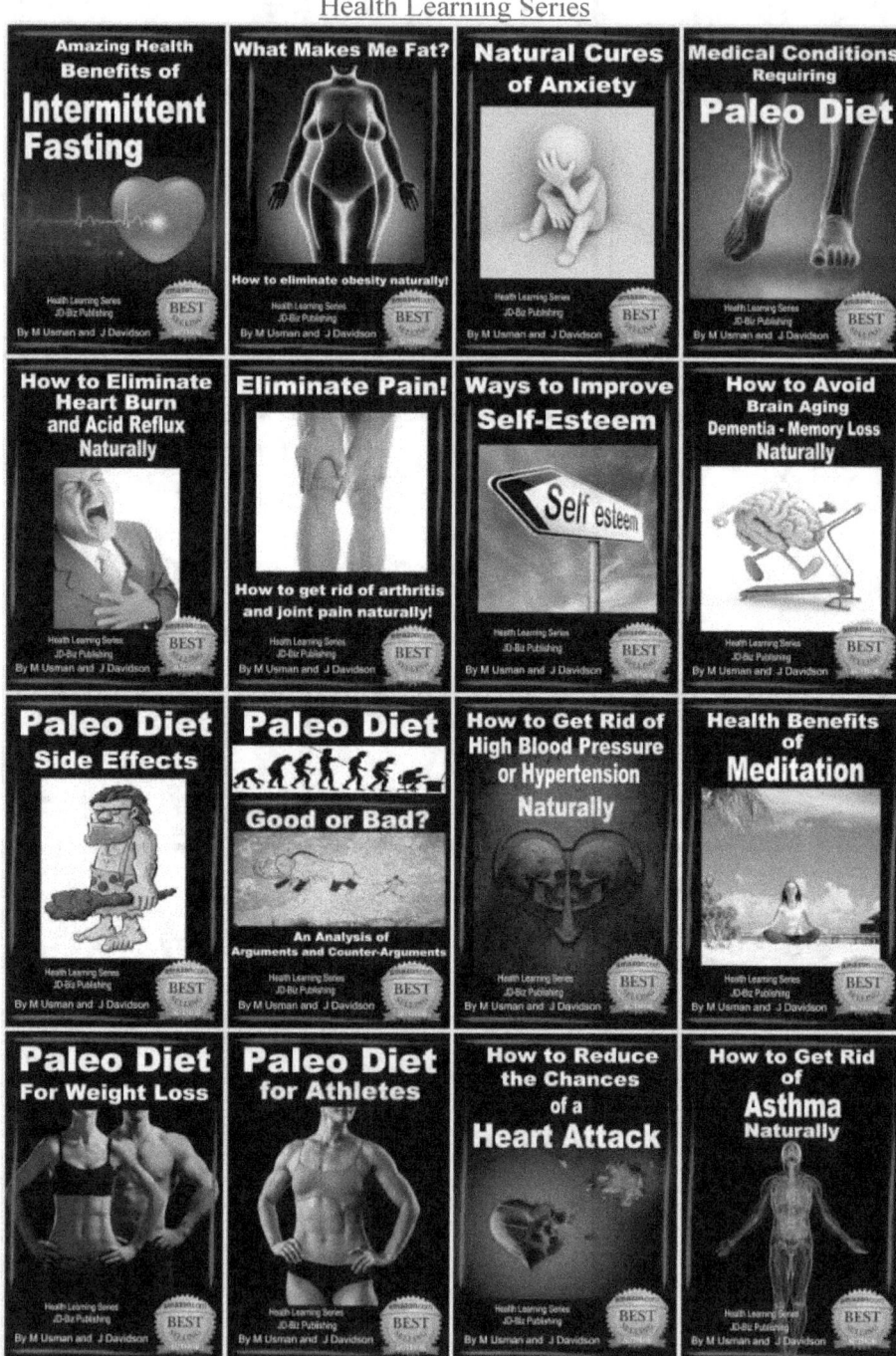

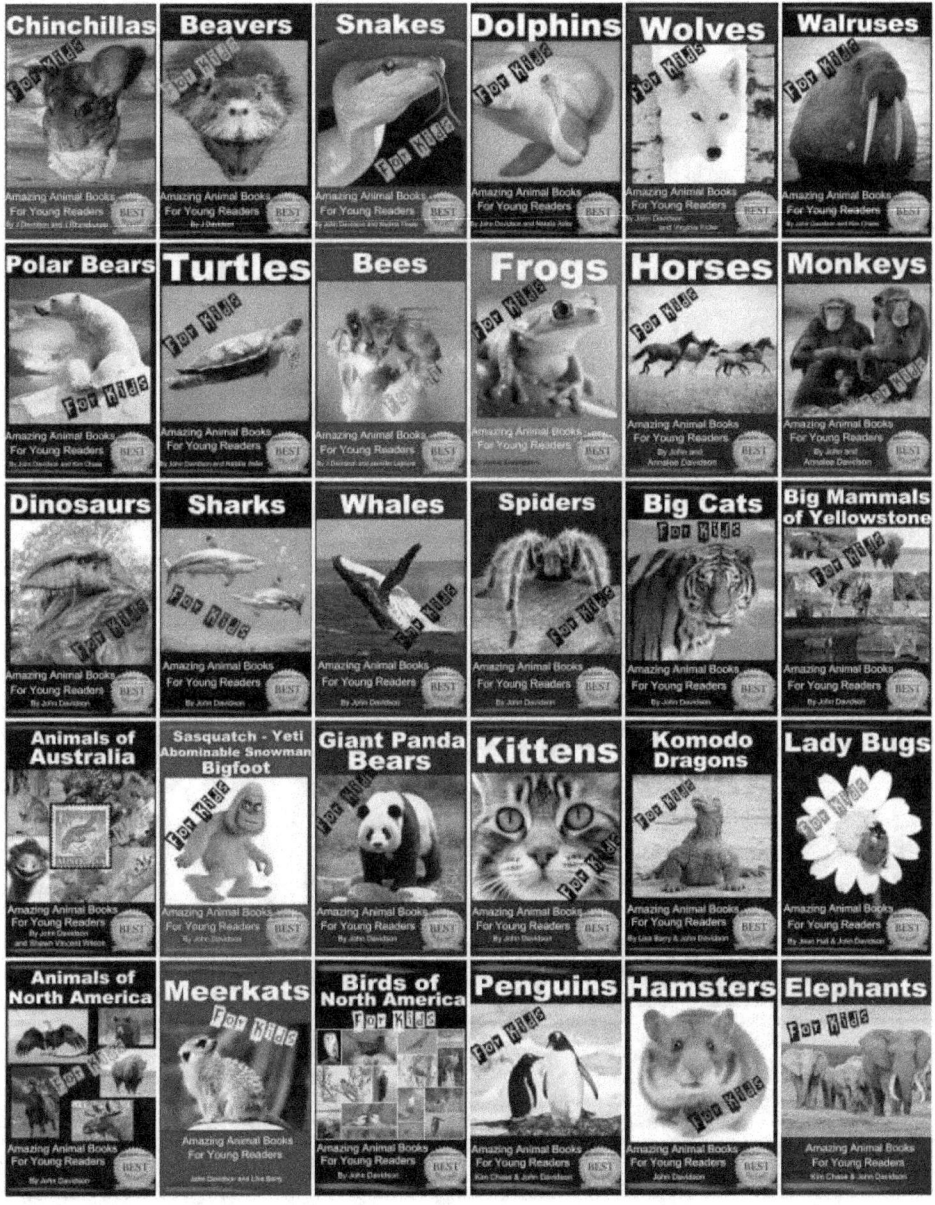

Learn To Draw Series

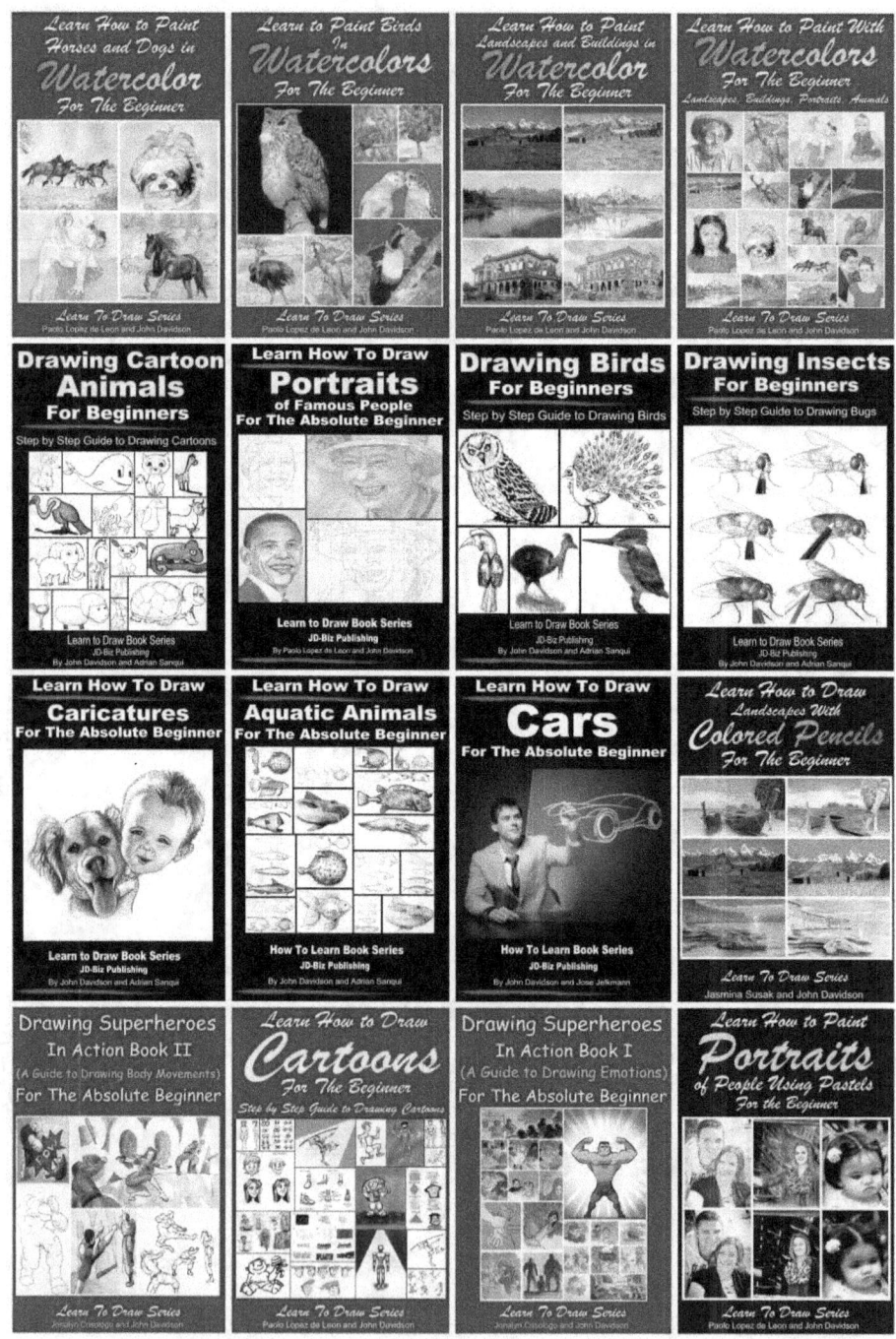

How to Build and Plan Books

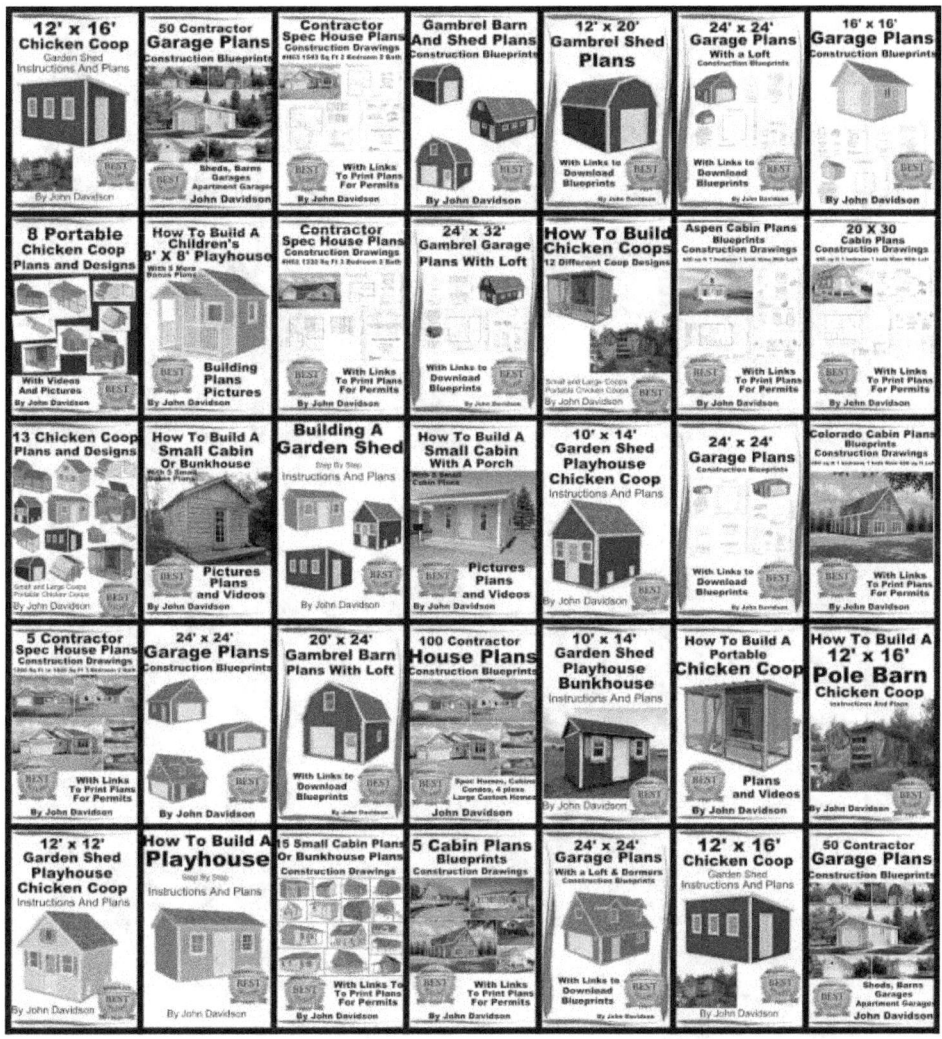

Entrepreneur Book Series

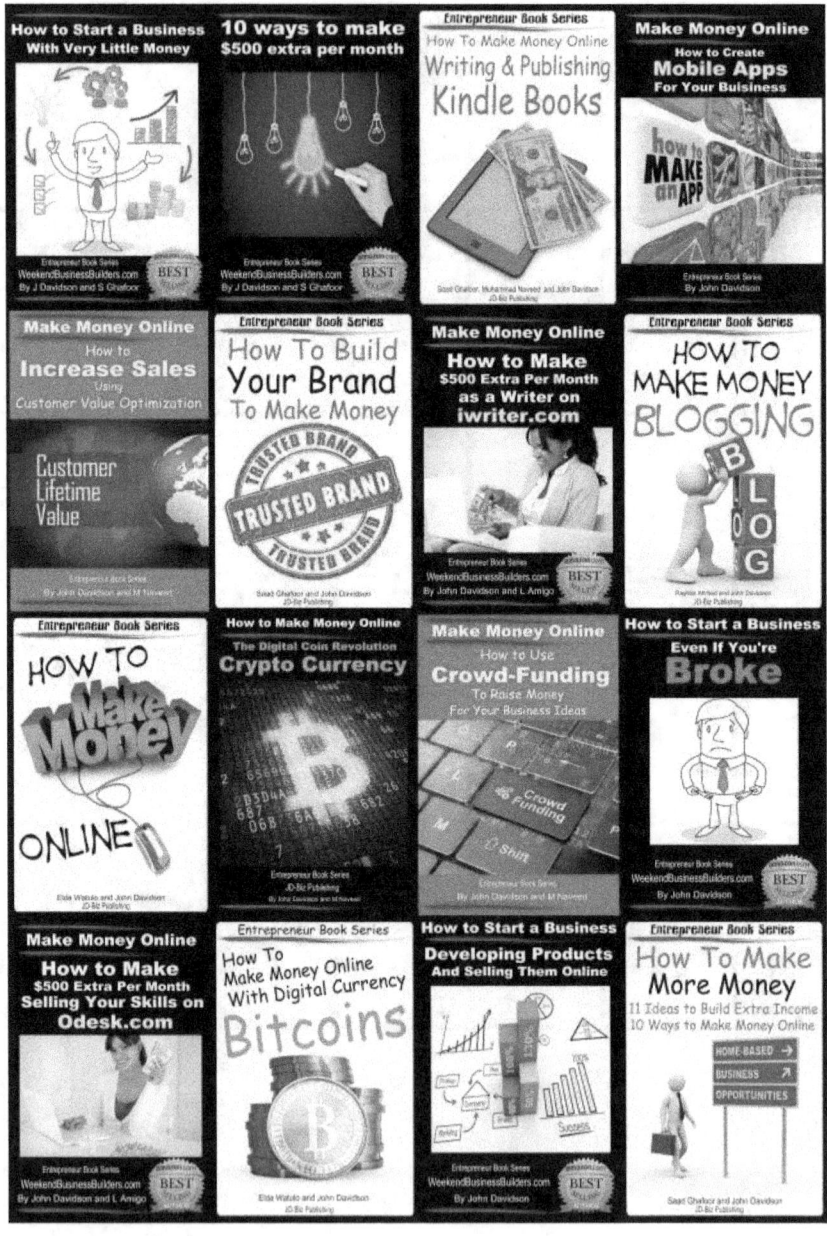

Our books are available at

1. Amazon.com

2. Barnes and Noble

3. Itunes

4. Kobo

5. Smashwords

6. Google Play Books

Publisher

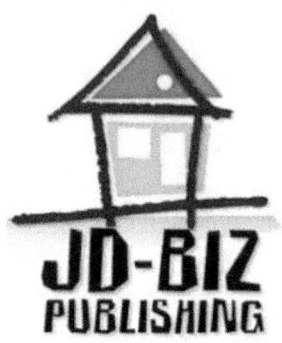

JD-Biz Corp

P O Box 374

Mendon, Utah 84325

http://www.jd-biz.com/

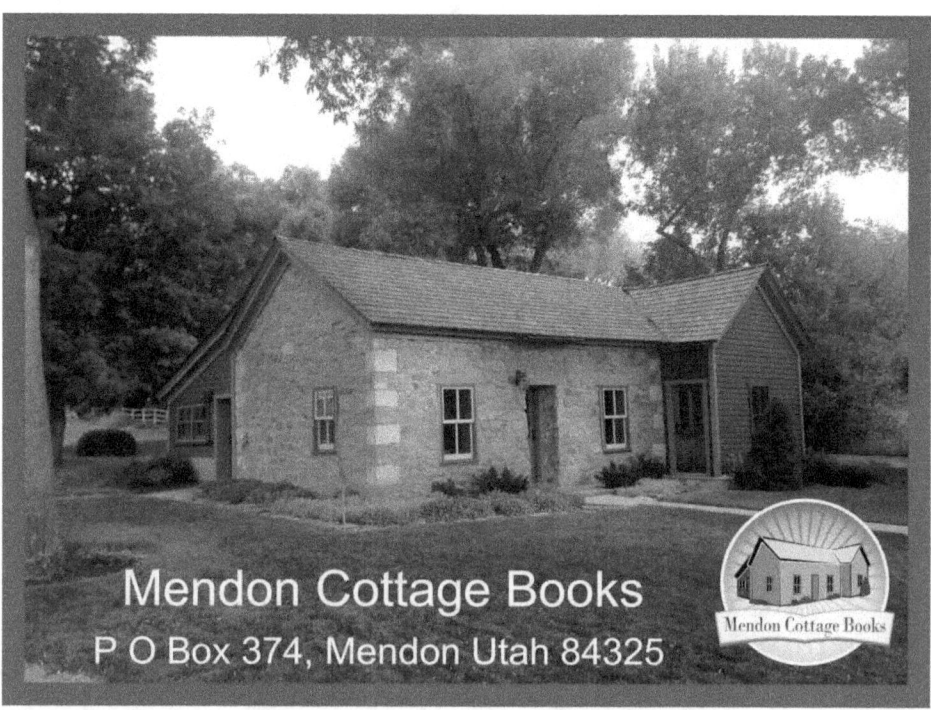

Mendon Cottage Books

P O Box 374, Mendon Utah 84325